I0476084

PSYCHIATRY IN THE SERVICE

OF MANKIND

A brief introduction to psychiatry and to the

help out there for people living with mental

illness, drug addiction and alcoholism

By Dr. M.E. Vijayasenan

This book is a brief introduction and general commentary on psychiatry. It does not, and should not replace the advice of a registered medical professional.

ISBN – 10: 1543025633

ISBN – 13: 978 - 1543025637

ABOUT THE AUTHOR

DR M.E VIJAYASENAN
B.Sc., M.B,B.S (MDS), D.I.H. (CAL), D.P.M.,
R.C.P., R.C.S. (LOND), M.R.C. PSYCH.
(LOND), F.R.A.N.Z.C.P. (NZ)

Dr Vijay, as he's known to his patients and colleagues, recently retired after spending the last 40 years working in New Zealand as a psychiatrist in both the public and private health systems. He occupied senior posts within the public system, opening a new psychiatric unit in one of the country's larger general hospitals where he served as Director of Psychiatric services. He was also directly involved in the training and development of young doctors training in the psychiatric field, and gains great satisfaction in seeing the success of his past students. He also developed his own private practice over many years, where he supported people with mental illness seeking help outside of the hospital system.

Inspired by his mother, herself a doctor, he began his career in medicine in India. He trained and qualified with a MBBS (Bachelor of Medicine, Bachelor of Surgery), later, specializing with a postgraduate diploma in Industrial Health, and went on to work for the Simpson Group Companies, a large multinational. While working there as a factory medical officer he noticed stress in some factory workers and helped them to cope with it. He later outlined the reasons for the stress in detail which resulted in difficulties both at work and in their personal lives, publishing his findings in the Indian Journal of Industrial Medicine.

Later when working in England he decided to pursue postgraduate study in psychiatry and attained membership to the Royal College of Psychiatrists in the United Kingdom.

Dr. Vijay is now a Fellow of the Royal Australian and New Zealand College of Psychiatrists.

Dr Vijay has always worked to improve the lives of his patients, showing great empathy and putting himself in someone's shoes when he worked with them.

CONTENTS

INTRODUCTION

This book is an easy to read and brief introductory narrative into psychiatry. It explores the fundamental premise of the body and mind working as one. I've included discussion on the identification and treatment of mental illness, as well as specifically looking at alcohol and drug dependence. Recently retired, I embarked on the process of putting some of the knowledge and experiences I gained into one place to share with anyone with an interest. Because it's always been my belief that knowledge not shared is knowledge wasted. This short book brings together my fifty years' experience working as a doctor, later specializing in psychiatry, in both public and private practice.

As a brief introduction and general commentary on psychiatry, this book can only touch the surface in what is a very detailed and varied field of study. I'll look in particular at the way our minds and bodies are intertwined and affect each other. And at the way mental illness is identified and treated, especially alcohol and drug dependence.

I was inspired to go into medicine by my mother, a doctor herself, who had a great care for the welfare of her patients, often providing free medical services for those unable to afford treatment. Like my mother, I treated my patients with empathy and compassion. In my career as a psychiatrist I worked to remove the stigma attached to mental illness and get the message to anyone affected by it to seek help. Just like physical illness can be treated, I believe mental illness can be too. And I point to the link often found between the two. My aim has always been to increase the avenues available for people with mental illness and make access to help easier.

In this book I emphasize the importance of psychiatry in medical treatment and the proper management of illnesses people experience. Advances in modern medicine show that all illnesses have areas of both physical suffering and mental stress. All major physical illnesses can create psychological issues. Many serious physical illnesses benefit from psychiatric assessment and help, as well as treatment for the physical symptoms. Where this happens, recovery is not only quicker, but better and longer lasting.

To put things very simply, when the body gets out of balance, this may result in physical illness. When the mind gets out of balance, conditions such as depression may occur. The great news is that, whether the problem is physical, mental or both, there's lots of help you can get by combining modern medical treatment with positive lifestyle changes. If you're coping with a health issue, or you're helping someone you know, you don't have to cope on your own. There is a path to recovery from depression, addictions to drugs and alcohol and other mental health issues. The first step is identifying there's a problem, the second is getting help.

As previously noted this is a brief introduction and general commentary on psychiatry. It does not, and should not, replace the advice of a registered medical professional. The diagnosis and treatment of any health condition is tailored for every individual, because everyone is different.

CHAPTER ONE - BODY AND MIND WORKING AS ONE

The World Health Organization defines health as "a state of complete physical, mental, and social well-being and not merely the absence of disease or infirmity."

You could say that the mind and body constantly react to each other and cannot be completely separated. Good medical practice stresses the treatment of the whole person, and not merely the particular disease someone may have. To do so effectively, a person's mental state needs to be taken into account as well as understanding the physical disease pattern. Someone's background, personality and environment is considered, as well the biological manner in which the person has adapted to things like pain, suffering, distress and fear.

In my early days of medical practice my mother showed me how many of the bodily illnesses which did not respond to prescribed drugs seemed to disappear miraculously once the underlying psychological factors were discovered. From this I ascertained that a good doctor understands that there is a mind as well as a body, and the two work in harmony. One is complementary to the other. They are delicately balanced and must be handled with the greatest care.

Let me explain this with extreme examples:

1. A patient with a certain type of brain tumor may initially not be physically sick and show symptoms of that tumor. They may however present with psychiatric symptoms like depression, anxiety and personality changes, with the symptoms of a brain tumor showing up very much latter. Understanding this particular psychiatric symptom enables the diagnosis of the condition early in order to save the patient.

2. Likewise there's the psychiatric illness Munchausen Syndrome, where someone seeks sympathy resulting in simulating and faking many physical illnesses. They often self-harm to the point of needing to be hospitalized. There's a subconscious presentation with symptoms simulating many physical illnesses. This is due to both conscious and unconscious mechanisms For example, a patient seeks attention by injuring their tongue or rectum with a knife or other sharp instrument, resulting in bleeding. They are secretly and purposefully play acting the symptoms, and causing genuine injury. This in turn may result in the person undergoing extensive medical and surgical investigations and treatments, including major

surgical procedures, without getting any visible benefit.

This clearly illustrates how it needs to be understood that the body and mind work in harmony, and the importance of identifying the underlying mental conditions when presented with a patient's physical illness to prevent any misdiagnosis.

3. Hypothyroidism (myxedema) is due to thyroid gland malfunction with patients complaining of puffy face, dry skin and cold intolerance. In addition, they have psychiatric symptoms of lethargy, anxiety, irritability, somatic delusions and hallucinations which can be used to diagnose the condition.

4. Pernicious anemia patients have physical symptoms such as weight loss, weakness and neuritis. They

also often experience mental issues such as depression with feelings of guilt and worthlessness.

It has always been my experience that the body and mind clearly work as one, and when I understood this, the benefits to my medical practice became obvious. These include early diagnosis of illnesses before physical symptoms display, as well as treatment of underlying mental issues resulting in reduction and sometimes elimination of physical symptoms that were previously not responding to prescribed drugs. For complete good health, it is my opinion that the mind and body need to operate in harmony.

CHAPTER TWO - THE HISTORY OF PSYCHIATRY FROM ANCIENT TIMES TO THE 21ST CENTURY

The wonderful thing about accumulating an immense body of knowledge from medicine and psychiatry throughout history is that we can preserve what is best, apply it in present day treatments, and discard what is no longer applicable.

The treatment of mental illness historically sometimes lacked compassion and understanding. Various activities like locking people up and confining them in dark rooms were practiced. There is a history of handling patients roughly, with the belief it would 'bring them to their senses'.

Hippocrates (460-355 B.C.) was describing depression among the Ancient Greeks as caused by increased humidity of the brain. When he believed it was due to an excess of black bile he named it melancholia. And if there was an excess of yellow bile as well, the melancholia might develop into mania. Even if we no longer put any faith in the 'four humors' theory today, this was one of the earliest pointers that mania and depression are connected, and forms part of the current diagnosis of bipolar disorder.

Since 2000 B.C possession by evil spirits had been thought to cause insanity in different parts of the world. During the Middle Ages, for example, people with mental illness were often regarded as witches that were possessed by evil spirits. Treatment for insanity often included practices such as exorcisms or even the burning of the body to save the soul. From these early times stigma and negatively stereotyping mental illness has a parallel history with this kind of 'unnatural' association.

Philippe Pinel was notable for his humane treatment of the mentally ill, particularly when he was appointed as chief of a large institution in Paris for custodial care in 1793. This indeed was progress, where people with a mental disorder were treated in a more compassionate way in what were then called asylums.

Following this, the number of asylums for the care of the mentally ill increased in the rest of the world, and this led in turn, to the development of clinical psychiatry. Many private and public mental asylums were built in Britain, from the year 1800. Many of these asylums used restraints in the form of handcuffs, straitjackets and chains. Later on, mechanical restraint was decreased throughout Britain, and this was replaced by appropriate medication that became available during that time. It has been alleged that mechanical restraint was replaced by chemical restraint to some extent.

In the late 18th century Franz Anton Mesmer practiced hypnotism, which he called an 'immense magnetism', and this has developed into modern day hypnosis to treat patients. J.M.Charcot the founder of modern neurology was appointed to the Chair in Diseases of the

Nervous System by the University of Paris in 1882, a position specially created for him. He was particularly interested in Hysteria with hypnotism as a form of treatment. As a result of his work there was greater acceptance and respectability of the subjects of neurology and psychotherapy. Later the French School of Neurologists and Psychotherapists produced outstanding psychiatrists, including Pierre Janet.

Sigmund Freud (1856-1939), who studied medicine and neurology, was interested in mild non-organic nervous disorders and tried to help patients with hypnosis. Later he developed the technique of psychoanalysis, in which the patient was encouraged to allow his thoughts to proceed without any conscious direction. He thought this unconscious process would reveal important discoveries about the patient, and assist in their recovery. By bringing this unconscious material into conscious mind, the patient would be relieved of his or her symptoms.

With the continuing development of treatments in psychiatry, the introduction of malariotherapy in 1917 was an important advancement in the history of psychiatry. Professor of Psychiatry Julius Wagner-Jauregg from Vienna, showed that inoculating a patient suffering from General Paresis of the Insane (or dementia paralytica) with malaria, could cure it. The malaria was then treated with quinine. He received a Noble Prize for this first successful treatment of mental disease by physical means, and raised great hopes for the future.

Sakel of Vienna introduced the treatment of Insulin Coma Therapy for patients suffering from withdrawal symptoms in drug addiction and published this as a success story in 1933. This treatment had a lot of support, but fell into disuse after the introduction of modern drugs like phenothiazine.

Electroconvulsive therapy was first introduced in 45 A.D. by a Roman physician, Scribonius Largus when he successfully treated people with mental illness by placing a Mediterranean torpedo fish across the brows of the sufferer. This fish was believed to generate the electric potential of 100 to 150 Volts. This was recorded as improving the mental health of the patients. Later in the 18th and 19th century this became the treatment of choice given to people who were suffering from insanity. Later the ECT treatment was perfected by a neuropsychiatrist, Ugo Cerletti, and was an effective treatment on many major psychiatric illnesses. ECT is still used in modern times for a few cases, but its use has declined with the availability of the modern psychotropic drugs.

In 1935 Egas Moniz persuaded his neurosurgical colleagues to destroy the connections of the frontal lobe of the brain in mentally ill patients who had marked anxiety. This did help to reduce the anxiety and their abnormal behavior, which helped these patients at that time. However since the introduction of modern psychotropic drugs this has been largely abandoned.

With modern effective medication and advanced psychiatric treatments, it's now possible to treat and help patients without the need to lock them away from society in asylums. Treatment can now be provided in hospitals and outpatient facilities like any other illness.

CHAPTER THREE - IDENTIFYING SYMPTOMS IN PSYCHIATRIC ILLNESS

When a person suffers symptoms of a disorder or disease, identifying the illness depends on identifying which part of the human function is being affected.

For example, someone developing a heart attack experiences a severe chest pain. We point to their cardiovascular system as the source of the problem. If someone develops pneumonia they often experience breathlessness, a severe cough and high fever. We say their respiratory system is affected.

Likewise, if someone experiences poor mental health, it affects the functions of their mind. While psychiatric illness can affect any part of the body, it most usually affects brain functions. And as with physical illnesses, it's possible to use evidence of how these functions of the mind are affected to identify different psychiatric conditions.

I'm going to divide up the functions of the mind like this:

1) Perception
2) Thought
3) Memory
4) Emotion and feeling
5) Consciousness
6) Intelligence and personality
7) Motor behavior

1. Disorders of perception

These consist of hallucinations and illusions.

a) Hallucinations

Hallucinations are where a person perceives something without an object. Or put another way, has a mental impression of sensory vividness without an adequate external stimulus. Hallucinations can affect any or all of the five human senses, affecting the functions of the eye and other sensors like smell, taste and tactile (feeling of being touched). For example, hearing voices and talking back to them when there is nobody there. We call these hallucinatory voices, and say the experience is an auditory hallucination.

Because these are disorders of perception, people are often not aware that there are no external stimuli producing the sensory reaction in their bodies. So they react to the false perception with an action. They are likely to feel that the action is appropriate in the circumstances, but to others nearby, it may appear to be bizarre behavior. This in turn may lead to bizarre interactions between the person experiencing hallucinations and the people around them.

Hallucinations can occur in many psychotic illnesses, including schizophrenia, drug abuse and alcohol abuse. In schizophrenia, a person might hear voices making derogatory comments about them without any people talking (auditory hallucination). Then the person with schizophrenia may think the voice making derogatory comments is coming from a person nearby, for example, and take an aggressive action.

Auditory hallucinations can also occur in delirium and organic physical disorders, such as when suffering from a high fever in influenza or typhoid.

b) Illusions

Illusions are when your senses become distorted when you are receiving actual stimuli. For example, there's a shadow in the room, but you genuinely see it as a person or a ghost. This is common in people experiencing anxiety and severe stress.

2. Disorders of Thought

Thought disorders can be considered as affecting the stream of thought, possession of thought and content of thought.

a) Streams of thought
The thought process is slowed down in depression, whereas in manic episodes the thoughts are pressured and speeded up into a flight of ideas.

In manic episodes the ideas follow in quick succession, with the train of thought determined by chance associations and 'clang' associations. Clang associations are characterized by grouping together words based on their sounds, such as using rhyming words even though the words themselves have no logical reason to be grouped together. Anxious and exhausted people may show a rather jerky train of thought.

Thought blocking is when the train of thought suddenly stops and a new one, totally unconnected with it, takes over. In schizophrenia there is evidence of thought blocking when the train of thought suddenly stops and a new one, totally unconnected with it takes over.

b) Possession of thought
- Obsessions

  Normally we experience our thoughts as belonging to us, and

we are in control of our thinking. With obsessive compulsive disorder, people experience the same thought that comes back to them, over and over again in a compulsive way. To the person's distress, they are unable to control and stop the thought repetition. These obsessive, ruminative thoughts may also become a part of an obsessive act. For example even though a person may have completed a task well, they doubt whether the task has been done correctly. This results in a repetition of this same task over and over again.

- Alienation of thought
This occurs in schizophrenia and can affect the thought process in several ways, including:

-Thought withdrawal –
someone experiences
their thoughts as being
taken away from their
mind by an outside
force over which they
have no control. They
may believe that some
other person takes their
thoughts with a definite
plan to use the ideas
from their mind.

-Thought insertion - the
person in distress
believes some new
thought, not their own,
is being inserted into
their mind. Usually
these are upsetting
vulgar thoughts, and get
the person very
distressed since they
cannot identify who is
doing it to them.

-Thought broadcasting - the person experiences that everyone else is participating in their thinking, and gets distressed since they wrongly believe others know what they are thinking.

All these experiences of thought alienation are first rank symptoms of schizophrenia and can help with identifying the condition.

c) Content of thought

Disorders of the content of thought are described as delusions. A delusion is an unshakable belief, despite being contradicted by reality. This arises from an internal disordered process, and is often a symptom used to identify a mental disorder. Delusions can be present in schizophrenia and other psychotic disorders including bipolar disorders.

Someone with schizophrenia experiencing auditory hallucination or the alienation of thought might be deluded that others are playing tricks on them, and may even act out violently against the person they think is responsible. This is called a paranoid delusion.

3. Disorders of Memory

We all forget things from time to time, like 'where did I leave my keys'. However indications that a person has a mental disorder is more than a simple lapse of memory.

When it has an effect on your daily life, work and social activities, then the memory loss may be indicative of a disorder or damage to the brain. The damage can occur a number of ways, such as physical injury, trauma of the brain or a stroke.

Memory loss is often a sign of dementia, especially in elderly patients. However, the symptoms may resemble memory loss caused from physical injury to the brain or a stroke, as described above. Even alcoholism and depression can cause symptoms that resemble dementia. This is why it is important to seek expert help, as a comprehensive evaluation is needed to identify whether or not dementia is present.

Other disorders of memory include Alzheimer's disease, where the loss of memory is gradual and progressive, also often associated with the elderly, and described as pre-senile dementia.

4. Disorders of emotion and feeling:

These are the emotional and mood changes which can occur in major depressive illness. Depressed people react emotionally to the usual concerns we all have, but in a more delusional way than normally expected. Concerns like our moral worth, bodily health, interpersonal relationships and material wealth and so on. Without any reality basis, they develop ideas of worthlessness and feelings of hopelessness, often together with suicidal ideas.

A person may believe that they suffer from a serious physical illness without actually having it, even when proved after full medical investigation. Their interpersonal relationships can be affected, since they may withdraw from all activities, including their usual hobbies. Their interest in sexual activity may decline, and the disorder can affect their physical libido. This may cause problems within intimate relationships, but I'm very pleased to say that once the loss of libido from major depression is successfully treated, a couple's joy and happiness often returns.

Delusions of low material worth with no reality basis may also develop. Major depression can result in the delusional belief that people are no good at anything, and can progress to such an extent that the sufferer develops delusions of low self-worth, followed by suicidal ideas and suicidal intent, to the extreme distress their family members. These emotional and mood changes can be used to identify major depression.

There can also be an elation of mood as in mania, with unwarranted cheerfulness coupled with a complete lack of insight.

Another disorder of emotion and feeling is anxiety, where people develop stress with a depressive mood. However they do not tend to become delusional, as in major depression.

With schizophrenia, a person may react inappropriately to the situation, which is described as incongruity of affect or emotion. For example, they may laugh at sad events or cry during happy occasions.

5. Consciousness

Consciousness is state of awareness of oneself and surroundings. When there is a disorder of the consciousness, symptoms include a lack of comprehension, attention and orientation to time and place. Disorders of consciousness can often result from a physical injury or trauma to the brain.

6. Intelligence and personality

Wechsler defines intelligence as 'the aggregate or global capacity of the individual to act purposely, to think rationally, and to deal effectively with his or her environment'. Changes in intelligence and personality can be symptomatic of an underlying mental or physical disorder.

People who are affected with changes to their intelligence and personality that are the result of a physical injury to the brain can exhibit abnormal behavior. More often than not, these disorders are a result of physical trauma rather than a psychiatric illness.

Long-term excess drug and alcohol consumption can also result in changes to intelligence and personality. In these cases medical and psychiatric intervention can be of great assistance and help.

7. Motor behavior

In psychiatric illnesses like bipolar disorder there are both manic and depressive states. When someone is manic there is excess of expressive movement, whereas there's a lack of it in depression. Obsessive compulsive disorder is sometimes wrongly regarded as a disorder of behavior. However, disturbed motor behavior is most often due to behavior disorders, rather than psychiatric illness.

While any of these symptoms may indicate that a psychiatric illness is present, it will benefit everyone to seek help and bring this to the attention of medical and psychiatric service providers. Modern psychiatry can definitely help identify if there is a psychiatric problem,

and if so, they are equipped to deal with these
very effectively.

CHAPTER FOUR - ALCOHOLISM
AND DRUG DEPENDENCE

Alcoholism

This term is used to designate heavy drinkers of all kinds, but can be broken down in the following ways:

1) Symptomatic Habitual Drinkers - they can stop when they want to.
2) Alcohol Addicts - who experience a loss of control. In other words, once they start drinking they cannot stop until they are too inebriated to drink any more, or become unconscious.
3) Alcoholics - show evidence of craving and alcohol withdrawal symptoms. They also show mental and physical changes due to alcohol.

The Development of Alcohol Addiction can be divided into three phases:

1. The Pre-alcoholic Phase - a person drinks to relieve the symptoms they experience due to the stresses of life. At first occasionally and later continuously.

2. The Crucial Phase - this begins with a loss of control. The phase progresses with the person drinking regularly and rationalizing their drinking behavior.

3. The Chronic Phase - this is when the person is regularly drinking both day and night, and they develop alcohol withdrawal symptoms when they are unable to get regular alcohol. Finally, all defenses fail. The person admits they are an alcoholic and goes on drinking.

There are psychological disorders associated with alcohol:

1) Pathological Intoxication

After taking a small quantity of alcohol some people develop a mild clouding of consciousness, together with very violent behavior. In this case the normal signs of drunkenness are absent. On recovery, people have no memory of the episode. Many of these people have abnormal EEG (Electro-Encephalogram - a recording of brain activity) records. This illness produces an organic twilight state in a susceptible person, due to excessive fluid intake and alcohol.

2) Delirium Tremens

This condition develops after many years of misuse of alcohol. However, due to injury or infection (for example) there may be a period of alcohol abstinence. It is this abstinence that is the causative factor of delirium tremens. This disorder is considered as a withdrawal phenomenon.

NB – People experiencing delirium tremens need hospital treatment, because they develop and experience withdrawal hyperarousal, visual hallucinations and seizures. They need urgent medical treatment.

3) Wernicke's Encephalopathy

This is due to acute bleeding in the brain due to a deficiency of thiamine (Vitamin B). This is due to poor diet and excessive vomiting together with dietary deficiencies created by alcoholism.

NB – People with Wernicke's encephalopathy need *urgent* treatment. Death often occurs, which is well documented in medical literature.

4) Alcoholic Korsakoff State

This illness is a form of alcohol-related brain injury characterized by a failure of the immediate memory, and is associated with polyneuritis. The memory loss is so severe that the individual tends to confabulate, which is a memory disturbance. The confabulation covers up gaps in the memory, where a person produces fabricated, distorted or misinterpreted memories without the intention to deceive. These people experience disorientation of time and place. They also have no insight into the disorder of their memory or the loss of orientation.

5) Alcoholic Dementia

Alcohol-related dementia is related to the excessive consumption of alcohol. This may come on slowly or follow delirium tremens, the Korsakoff state or Wernicke's encephalopathy.

6) Alcoholic Diminished sexual function

Diminished sexual functioning due to alcohol has been described by various authors. India's most famous and probably the oldest treatise on the art of love, the Kamasutra, talks of Kama, the enjoyment of objects with the help of the five senses. It explains how these senses get impaired by consuming Mathu (alcohol) and other intoxicants.

No one has improved on Shakespeare`s observation of the sexual effects of alcohol -"It provokes and unprovokes: it provokes the desire, but it takes away the performance" (Macbeth, Act2, Scene-3). Nearly 400 years later, we are beginning to learn that not only the acute, but also chronic excessive ingestion of alcohol has a profound and complex effect on sexual function.

7) Paranoid reactions and developments

These can be described as delusions where, without reality basis, someone has a strong belief and also reacts accordingly. While in this delusional state, people believe they are having an understandable reaction. In their own mind, the interaction of their personality with the environment is correct and justifiable. Morbid jealousy is a common paranoid development in chronic alcoholism, where the person has the delusion that their spouse is being unfaithful. It can occur in either sex, but appears more common in men, so it's often called 'jealous husband syndrome' or the `Othello syndrome`.

Drug Addiction

There are three main groups of drugs, grouped according to their pharmacological effects.

1. Opiates - morphine, heroin, pethidine and other synthetic drugs.
2. Euphoriants - cocaine, cannabis, along with the sympathomimetic amines and the hallucinogenic group of drugs.
3. Hypnotics - barbiturates and hypnotic drugs.

1)   Opiate addiction

All the analgesic drugs can cause physical dependence and emotional dependence. If morphine is taken for non-medical reasons it can cause nausea, vomiting and malaise at first. But after repeatedly taking the drug, the person drifts off into a light sleep and then wakes up and nods off repeatedly, with constant drowsiness. During the drowsiness, there is a feeling of serenity and happiness.

Intravenous administration of this drug produces dizziness, flushing, itching and a rumbling in the stomach. A sensation occurs in the abdomen like an orgasm, but it does not affect the genitals.

Symptoms of drug addiction to opiates
    The pupils are constricted and constipation is always present.

50

Once the person develops a dependence on a drug like opium, they develop a withdrawal syndrome when it is not available. Look out for the following symptoms:

- Yawning
- Perspiration
- Absolute insomnia
- Muscular twittering,
- Hot and cold flushes,
- Retching and vomiting where urgent medical care and treatment is required.

2) Euphoriant addiction

Cocaine

This is taken as snuff, or intravenously. It produces an ecstatic sensation of extreme mental and physical power, with the abolition of all sensation of fatigue and hunger. If this substance is taken for a longer period, a paranoid psychosis develops, which needs urgent medical and psychiatric help.

Cannabis

This substance is usually smoked and produces elation and distortion of space and time. Cannabis does not cause physical addiction but can result in emotional dependence.

Dextroamphetamine and Methamphetamine

When taken, these substances produce euphoria with grandiose ideas, inexhaustibility and impaired judgement. When taken for a long period they induce a paranoid psychosis indistinguishable from schizophrenia.

3) Hypnotics addiction

Barbiturates and other hypnotic drugs are prescribed by doctors for various medical illnesses such as bipolar disorder (to control mood swings) and to epileptic people (to control seizures). They are also used to assist with the sleep difficulties that occur with various medical and psychiatric illnesses. Caution is needed, however, because people taking these drugs can develop a tolerance to the barbiturates and become addicted. Usually doctors treat their patients by prescribing the minimal dose required, and never encourage increasing the dose.

Once a drug or alcohol dependence is suspected in an individual, medical and psychiatric help should be sought, as well as the support of family and friends.

CHAPTER FIVE - THE TREATMENT AND MANAGEMENT OF PSYCHIATRIC DISORDERS

General Principles of helping people with a psychiatric disorder

After completing a medical degree, a doctor can undergo further training to specialize in psychiatry. They are trained to understand that the most important aspect of helping any patient is to have empathy with them. In other words, to properly understand a patient's suffering, a doctor should put themselves in their shoes to recognize how they feel.

By doing this, a psychiatrist can better understand the difficulties someone is going through. Every effort has to be made to put the person at ease and create a feeling of true sympathy, which enables them to talk about their problems and difficulties freely. The art of interviewing can only be learned by experience.

In psychiatry, it's not only the assessment of the patient that's important. Consideration should also be taken of their relationship with their family, together with the environment they are exposed to. After this assessment a more complete diagnosis can be made.

The psychiatric diagnosis covers five aspects:
1. The main psychiatric illness
2. The patient's personality
3. Any details of coexisting physical illness
4. The extent of suffering
5. The extent of environmental stress and support, together with a measure of the present stress and suffering.

Psychiatric Treatment

Psychiatric treatment includes not only treating the patient but also their family. This helps the family to better understand the patient and provide support to them. The psychiatric treatment team can consist of the psychiatrist together with nurses, psychologists, social workers, occupational therapists and sometimes an alcohol drug addiction councilor.

Drugs and psychotherapy

Psychiatric illnesses are usually treated with drugs and psychotherapy. Certain psychiatric illnesses respond only to drugs, while some others benefit more with psychotherapy. Some mental illnesses respond best to a combination of both.

A drug used for psychiatric illness has the same effect on different cultural groups all over the world. On the other hand, for psychotherapy to be effective, it has to take a different approach to accommodate the features and aspects of different cultures.

East and west

Many psychiatrists from the East, including those from India, have reported that the classical stages of personality development as described by Freud and the post-Freudians, have limited applications in their own societies. For example, the role of fathers as exemplified in the Oedipus complex can be very different in a non-European culture.

In Eastern culture, the concept of dependency has quite different connotations from those associated with it in Europe and America. In the west, dependency is seen as an attribute of immaturity which would be outgrown when the individual reaches adulthood. But in the East, it is accepted as a continuing trait, that is manifested in certain relationships, and can carry on well into old age.

The Western emphasis on individual autonomy is also alien to Eastern ways of thinking. Consequently, a patient from an Eastern culture does not necessarily feel at ease when offered the detached impersonal guidance of Western-oriented psychotherapy. Instead he or she requires their psychiatrist to assume the role of a

Guru or idealized father-figure and expects to receive the Guru's guidance and support in his or her search for their personal solutions.

Multicultural New Zealand

In my opinion there will, in time, be many variants of psychotherapy to accommodate different cultures. At present, there are so many cultural exchanges in so many spheres that it should be feasible to trade information, new techniques and methodologies in the treatment of mental illness as well. In the future, this should bring a lot of benefit to people experiencing mental illness, no matter which culture they belong to. As a multicultural society, I believe New Zealand can lead the way in the world to help everyone affected by mental illness, addiction and alcohol abuse.

CONCLUSION

After over 45 years in the psychiatric profession, I am heartened by the improving awareness, understanding and attitude towards those with mental health issues. This has been possible as a result of the hard work of mental health professionals to make it easier for those seeking help to get it. Public awareness campaigns that include high profile people such as sporting celebrities talking about their mental health issues in the public arena, have helped reduce the stigma attached. This combined with publicity of places to seek help and telephone helplines has made it easier to get effective and timely help and treatment.

Today people that have a psychiatric set back find it easier to seek help as a result of the reduced stigma attached to mental health issues and can be effectively treated with modern psychiatric help. There have been great strides and advancements in psychiatry with better diagnostic facilities and customised treatments right from the initial assessment. There are now increased resources and understanding about psychiatric illness, with modern drugs together with holistic treatments like family therapy, occupational therapy and social support where environmental factors of the patient are taken into consideration when designing a treatment plan. A complete treatment plan also includes regular follow ups once patients improve.

Psychiatrists are now well trained in the understanding of psychiatric illness and also in general medicine and can work closely with other hospital specialists as a coordinated team. They can help to treat patients in general hospitals, who at times have both a significant medical illness as well as a psychiatric disorder. In modern general hospitals there is a liaison psychiatrist working closely with other hospital specialists so that when required both body and mind is taken into account while treating people. Following treatment, people can regain their quality of life and pursue the same activities they engaged in prior to the set back.

GLOSSARY

Analgesic

Analgesia means inability to feel pain. Drugs used to reduce pain are called as analgesics.

Anxiety

An unpleasant affective state with the expectation, but not the certainty, of something unpleasant happening.

Barbiturates

A derivative of barbituric acid, such as baritones or phenobarbitone, used in medicine as a sedative or hypnotic.

Bipolar disorder

A brain disorder, characterised by two opposed shifts in mood or energy. For example, depression with feelings of dejection which colours all thought and activity at times, changing into a state of marked cheerfulness associated with infectious gaiety in mania.

Blackout

Loss of consciousness or loss of memory.

Brain tumour

A growth of abnormal cells in the brain, or close to the brain, that multiplies in an uncontrollable way. 70% of patients with brain tumours have psychological disorders. These can be classified as:

> 1) Clouding of consciousness, with 38% of patients showing psychological symptoms.
>
> 2) Severe headaches.
>
> 3) The amnestic syndrome. This is a subacute organic psychiatric state in which the presenting features are difficulties in registering new memories, confabulation and complete disorientation of time and place. Comprehension is disordered and there is a 'tram-line` or linear thinking.

Clang association

Two thoughts are associated on the basis of rhyme or assonance

Compulsion

An act which a person feels compelled to carry out, although he or she realizes that it is senseless.

Confabulation

Detailed false memories.

Conscious and Sub-consciousness

This is made up of personal and collective parts of awareness. The conscious mind is the part responsible for logic and reasoning and controls the actions you choose to do. For example, if you calculate how much change you should receive when you hand over one dollar for a sixty cent purchase, or decide to throw a ball or lift an object, it is the conscious mind that enables the action.

The subconscious mind on the other hand operates outside of the conscious mind and is the part responsible for the involuntary actions we do, such as our eyes blinking through the day.

Thought processes in the personal sub-conscious are often the reverse of those in the conscious mind. The shadow is the reverse of those in the conscious mind, comprising all the emotional aspects of the conscious psyche. This is partly collective, as well as personal.

Delirium

An acute organic state in which consciousness is changed in a dream-like way.

Delusion

An unshakable belief which is out of keeping with the person's educational, cultural and social background.

Dementia

A permanent loss of intellectual function due to coarse brain disease. If it occurs before senility due to injury to the brain or other disorder like

Alzheimer's disease. It is called pre-senile dementia. Setbacks in old age are called senile dementia.

Depression

An emotional state of mind characterized by feelings of gloom and inadequacy, leading to withdrawal.

Drug addiction

A psychological or physical dependence on the effects of a drug, which leads to an overpowering need for the drug and to obtaining it by any means.

Electro Convulsive Treatment (ECT)

An epileptic fit produced by the passage of an electric current through the head by means of electrodes applied to the temples.

EEG (Electro-encephalogram)

An instrument used to record brain electrical activity in a graph, usually by means of electrodes placed on the scalp. It is used to study brain waves and also to diagnose tumors of the brain.

Euphoriants

A drug which induces euphoria, which is a persistent elevation of mood, usually associated with a sense of bodily wellbeing.

Flight of ideas

A rapid progress of thought in which the individual elements are not rationally connected, but where their sequence depends on chance associations particularly on rhyming and assonance (see also Clang associations).This characteristically occurs in mania.

Hallucination

A perception without an external object.

Hypnotics

Drugs used to induce sleep. These drugs are prescribed for a short period only. These drugs are useful, but patients can develop tolerance and become addicted.

Hysteria

A mental illness in which the brain and nervous systems are unconsciously motivated.

Hypnosis

An artificially induced state of semi-consciousness, characterised by an increased suggestibility to the words of a hypnotist. This is used clinically to reveal unconscious memories.

Libido

Generally used to describe sexual desire and sexual drive.

Mania

A mental illness characterised by elevated mood, flight of ideas and over activity.

Melancholia

A mental state characterised by depression and irrational fears.

Motor behavior

Obsessions and compulsions can be regarded as disorders of this kind, since the normally subjective experience of the progress of thought and action is disturbed.

Nervous system

The sensory and control apparatus of humans consisting of networks of nerve cells including the brain and the spinal cord.

Neurology

The study of the anatomy, physiology and the diseases of the nervous system.

Opiates

Any of the narcotic drugs containing opium or an alkaloid opium. It induces sedation and sleep. Regular use can cause addiction.

Obsession

A content of consciousness which you cannot get rid of, although when it occurs it is judged to be a senseless or dominating without a cause.

The essential feature is that this experience occurs against the person's will but it is recognised as his or her own thoughts.

Withdrawal Syndrome – Alcohol & Drugs

In drug and alcohol addiction there is a physical change in the nervous system so that normal functions cannot continue without an adequate intake of the drug or alcohol. If the drugs or alcohol are withdrawn, symptoms appear which are due to the malfunctioning of the nervous system. These symptoms constitute the withdrawal symptoms which may last for hours or days depending the nature of the drug or the individual's constitution.